DIABETIC COOKBOOK GUIDE FOR BEGINNERS

DIABETIC-FRIENDLY RECIPE DISHES FOR EACH MEAL TYPE

Table of Contents

Introduction

Diabetes is not new to all of us. We have probably heard of a friend, a family member or an officemate who has this chronic disease. It is a health condition wherein the individual has a blood sugar level that is beyond normal.

Of course, this book will not be complete without telling you about the foods to you should avoid and eat. Diet is very important in Diabetes management that is why in Chapter 3 you will see some tips on how to balance your meals.

There are a lot of ways to control your blood sugar levels. Every individual is unique; thus, everyone has different ways of facing this health condition. But in this book, for sure you will be able to find one or most of them effective. It will be to your benefit to try them all and see for yourself which among them is most suited for you.

In this book, you will learn so many things about diabetes, blood sugar levels, and how to keep your sugar level in control.

This book aims to inspire, give hope and inform people that it is never too late to make the necessary changes in your diet and lifestyle so you could better manage your health condition. We just need to take matters into our own hands and do what is necessary to avoid further complications and stay healthy. There will be tips on having the proper mindset, meal planning, and other lifestyle changes.

Again, I want to thank you for purchasing this book. I hope this will be the beginning of your healthy life.

Enjoy reading and learning!

Types of Diabetes

In this diabetic cookbook, we revealed four (4) types of Diabetes – Type 1 diabetes, Type 2 diabetes, Gestational diabetes, and Prediabetes. Now, let us discuss the different types of diabetes in detail.

Type 1 Diabetes

You may have heard of this type of diabetes as "adolescent" diabetes, as it usually occurs in children and young adults. But type 1 diabetes is uncommon because it occurs in only 5-10% of diabetic patients.

You see, no matter the challenges you have had with type 1 diabetes, you can now take your health back by balancing your diets, medications, and exercises. Also, you can discuss your health conditions with family members, friends, and associates who live with type 1 diabetes as well. Below, we highlight three effective ways to manage type 1 diabetes.

Coping With Type 1 Diabetes

Although we have different methods to manage type 1 diabetes, the most effective way is to work closely with your health care provider. So, whenever your doctor diagnosed you with type 1 diabetes, you need to pay attention to the following things to live healthier.

1. Manage Your Medication: Always seek medical attention, and learn the best way to test your blood sugar level without a needle using a device like; OneTouch Ultra Mini Blood Glucose Monitoring System. Don't result to self-help or make any major

change in diet and lifestyle without consulting with your healthcare provider. You should understand that being a diabetic, makes your life fragile like a piece of glass. So, you must be mindful of what you eat, drink, and engage in. This is because a minor change in diet and lifestyle can cause severe damage or loss of life in most cases. Hence, you can't afford to live anyhow, just like everyone does.

2. Eat Well To Live Well: Honestly, it is challenging and a bit frustrating to select the class of food to eat as a type 1 diabetic patient. This is because there is no general rule to handpick safe food for diabetic patients. Remember, everyone's body is not the same. You might be allergic to certain foods found on the diabetic approved food list, making it hard to choose what to eat and what not to eat. Ideally, foods that can lower blood sugar levels are all considered safe for type 1 diabetic patients. The rules for making the right choices are to experiment with the foods you eat and consult with your healthcare provider as well. Watch how your body reacts after eating foods you are not familiar with and adjust. Start small, and if the food affects your body negatively, quit it. Above all, monitor your blood glucose at home to ensure you are safe.

3. Avoid Unhealthy Lifestyle: Certain unhealthy habits like stress, physical inactivities, smoking, obesity, or being overweight can increase your risk of diabetes. Cutting down on things that lead to depression and anxiety is the best way to overcome type 1 diabetes. This is because depression and anxiety are among the

symptoms of type 1 diabetes. So, pay attention to your mental health so you can live healthier and longer.

Type 2 Diabetes

This type of diabetes is most common in 90-95% of all type 2 diabetes. In common terms, we can say that type 2 diabetes is a life-threatening disease that causes your blood sugar to be higher than normal. In type 2 diabetes, your pancreas or cells no longer makes enough insulin, or respond to insulin all. But, no matter what, your life does not end with type 2 diabetes — Whether you are newly diagnosed with type 2 diabetes or you have been living with it for a long time, you can get back your health on track following a healthy lifestyle, eating well, and coupled with doctor's prescription.

As a diabetic patient, you cannot ignore the importance of diet, weight loss, and exercise in your routine. At the moment, there is no cure for type 2 diabetes, hence, weight loss, healthy eating plans, and exercises can help to manage your health, and if this does not produce the required results, your doctor may prescribe oral medications.

Coping Mechanisms to Reverse Type 2 Diabetes

1. Get a blood sugar logbook so you can test and record your blood sugar readings.

2. Open up and discuss with others who have type 1 or type 2 diabetes

3. Manage your stress level

4. Eat more non-starchy vegetables, salmon, whole grains, and fruits.

5. Monitor early signs of diabetes; such as frequent urination, blurred vision, swelling in feet and ankles, dizziness, increased thirst, itching, and yeast infection.

6. In an emergency, learn to give yourself insulin by syringe, pen, or pump.

Gestational Diabetes

Gestational diabetes occurs in most women during pregnancy, and it typically affects 2-7% of all pregnancies in the United States. It is caused by the inability of your pancreas to deliver insulin to control glucose levels in your body. Essentially, this form of diabetes disappears after pregnancy. But there is an increased risk that both mother and child might develop type 2 diabetes soon. So, doctors usually test for gestational diabetes on/before the 26th week of pregnancy and might recommend certain healthy diets, exercises, and insulin injections. Now, see the list below of how to prevent and cope with gestational diabetes.

Recipes

Breakfast

1 Sweet Pancakes

Preparation Time: 10 minutes

Cooking Time: 5 minutes

Servings: 5

Ingredients:

All-purpose flour – 1 cup

Granulated sugar – 1 Tablespoon

Baking powder – 2 teaspoons.

Egg whites – 2

Almond milk - 1 cup

Olive oil - 2 Tablespoons.

Maple extract – 1 Tablespoon

Directions:

Combine the flour, sugar and baking powder in a bowl.

Make a well in the center and place to one side.

Mix the egg whites, milk, oil, and maple extract, do this in another bowl.

Add the egg mixture to the well and gently mix until a batter is formed.

Heat skillet over medium heat.

Cook 2 minutes on each side or until the pancake is golden only add 1/5 of the batter to the pan.

Repeat with the remaining batter and serve.

Nutrition:

Calories: 178

Fat: 6g

Potassium: 126mg

Sodium: 297mg

Protein: 6g

2 Breakfast Smoothie

Preparation Time: 15 minutes

Cooking Time: 0 minute

Servings: 2

Ingredients:

Frozen blueberries – 1 cup

Pineapple chunks – ½ cup

English cucumber – ½ cup

Apple – ½

Water – ½ cup

Directions:

Put the pineapple, blueberries, cucumber, apple, and water in a blender and blend until thick and smooth.

Pour into 2 glasses and serve.

Nutrition:

Calories: 87

Fat: g

Carb: 22g

Phosphorus: 28mg

Potassium: 192mg

Sodium: 3mg

Protein: 0.7g

3 Buckwheat and Grapefruit Porridge

Preparation Time: 5 minutes

Cooking Time: 20 minutes

Servings: 2

Ingredients:

Buckwheat – ½ cup

Grapefruit – ¼, chopped

Honey – 1 Tablespoon

Almond milk – 1 ½ cups

Water – 2 cups

Directions:

Boil water on the stove. Add the buckwheat and place the lid on the pan.

Simmer for 7 to 10 minutes, in a lowheat. Check to ensure water does not dry out.

Remove and set aside for 5 minutes, do this when most of the water is absorbed.

Drain excess water from the pan and stir in almond milk, heating through for 5 minutes.

Add the honey and grapefruit.

Serve.

Nutrition:

Calories: 231

Fat: 4g

Carb: 43g

Phosphorus: 165mg

Potassium: 370mg

Sodium: 135mg

4 Egg and Veggie Muffins

Preparation Time: 15 minutes

Cooking Time: 20 minutes

Servings: 4

Ingredients:

Cooking spray

Eggs – 4

Unsweetened rice milk – 2 Tablespoon

Sweet onion – ½, chopped

Red bell pepper – ½, chopped

Pinch red pepper flakes

Pinch ground black pepper

Directions:

Preheat the oven to 350F.

Spray 4 muffin pans with cooking spray. Set aside.

Whisk together the milk, eggs, onion, red pepper, parsley, red pepper flakes, and black pepper until mixed.

Pour the egg mixture into prepared muffin pans.

Bake until the muffins are puffed and golden, about 18 to 20 minutes.

serve

Nutrition:

Calories: 84

Fat: 5g

Carb: 3g

Phosphorus: 110mg

Potassium: 117mg

Sodium: 75mg

Protein: 7g

5 Cherry Berry Bulgur Bowl

Preparation Time: 15 minutes

Cooking Time: 15 minutes

Servings: 4

Ingredients:

1 cup medium-grind bulgur

2 cups water

Pinch salt

1 cup halved and pitted cherries or 1 cup canned cherries, drained

½ cup raspberries

½ cup blackberries

1 tablespoon cherry jam

2 cups plain whole-milk yogurt

Directions:

Mix the bulgur, water, and salt in a medium saucepan. Do this in a medium heat. Bring to a boil.

Reduce the heat to low and simmer, partially covered, for 12 to 15 minutes or until the bulgur is almost tender. Cover, and let stand for 5 minutes to finish cooking do this after removing the pan from the heat.

While the bulgur is cooking, combine the raspberries and blackberries in a medium bowl. Stir the cherry jam into the fruit.

When the bulgur is tender, divide among four bowls. Top each bowl with ½ cup of yogurt and an equal amount of the berry mixture and serve.

Nutrition:

Calories: 242;

Total fat: 6g

Saturated fat: 3g

Sodium: 85mg

Phosphorus: 237mg

Potassium: 438mg

Carbohydrates: 44g

Fiber: 7g

Protein: 9g

Sugar: 13g

6 Baked Curried Apple Oatmeal Cups

Preparation Time: 10 minutes

Cooking Time: 20 minutes

Servings: 6

Ingredients:

3½ cups old-fashioned oats

3 tablespoons brown sugar

2 teaspoons of your preferred curry powder

⅛ teaspoon salt

1 cup unsweetened almond milk

1 cup unsweetened applesauce

1 teaspoon vanilla

½ cup chopped walnuts

Directions:

Preheat the oven to 375°F. Then spray a 12-cup muffin tin with baking spray then set aside.

Combine the oats, brown sugar, curry powder, and salt, and mix in a medium bowl.

Mix together the milk, applesauce, and vanilla in a small bowl,

Stir the liquid ingredients into the dry ingredients and mix until just combined. Stir in the walnuts.

Using a scant ⅓ cup for each divide the mixture among the muffin cups.

Bake this for 18 to 20 minutes until the oatmeal is firm. Serve.

Nutrition: For 2 Oatmeal Cups:

Calories: 296;

Total fat: 10g

Saturated fat: 1g

Sodium: 84mg

Phosphorus: 236mg

Potassium: 289mg

Carbohydrates: 45g

Fiber: 6g

Protein: 8g

Sugar: 11g

7 Pumpkin Bread

Preparation Time: 10 Minutes

Cooking Time: 50 Minutes

Servings: 12

Ingredients:

¾ cup Pumpkin Puree

¼ cup Pumpkin Seeds

2 cups Almond Flour, blanched

1/3 cup Butter

½ cup Coconut Flour

4 Eggs, large

¾ cup Erythritol

¼ tsp. Sea Salt

2 tsp. Baking Powder

2 tsp. Pumpkin Spice

Directions:

Preheat the oven to 350° F.

Mix all the dry ingredients in a large mixing bowl until combined well.

In another bowl, beat together eggs, pumpkin puree and melted butter with a whisker until combined.

Transfer the batter to a parchment paper-lined so that the paper hangs over the sides. Smoothen the top and garnish it with pumpkin seeds.

Bake for 55 to 60 minutes or until a toothpick inserted in the center comes clean.

Allow it to cool for some time before slicing.

Tip: Serve it along with cream cheese.

Nutrition: Calories: 215Kcal Carbohydrates: 4g Proteins: 8g Fat: 18g Sodium: 147g

---

Meat Mains

8 Chicken Soup

Preparation time: 10 minutes

Cooking time: 30 minutes

Servings: 6

Ingredients:

4 lbs. Chicken, cut into pieces

5 carrots, sliced thick

8 cups of water

2 celery stalks, sliced 1 inch thick

2 large onions, sliced

Directions:

In a large pot add chicken, water, and salt. Bring to boil.

Add celery and onion in the pot and stir well.

Turn heat to medium-low and simmer for 30 minutes.

Add carrots and cover pot with a lid and simmer for 40 minutes.

Remove Chicken from the pot and remove bones and cut Chicken into bite-size pieces.

Return chicken into the pot and stir well.

Nutrition: Calories: 89 Fat: 6.33gCarbohydrates: 0g Protein: 7.56g Sugar: 0gCholesterol: 0mg

9 Roasted Pork

Preparation time: 10 minutes

Cooking time: 30 minutes

Servings: 5

Ingredients:

500-2000g Pork meat (To roast)

Salt

Oil

Directions:

Join the cuts in an orderly manner.

Place the meat on the plate

Varnish with a little oil.

Place the roasts with the fat side down.

Cook in air fryer at 1800C for 30 minutes.

Turn when you hear the beep.

Remove from the oven. Drain excess juice.

Let stand for 10 minutes on aluminum foil before serving.

Nutrition: Calories: 820 Fat: 41g Carbohydrates: 0g Protein: 20.99g Sugar: 0gCholesterol: 120mg

10   Marinated Loin Potatoes

Preparation time: 10 minutes

Cooking time: 30 minutes

Servings: 2

Ingredients:

2 medium potatoes

4 fillets of marinated loin

A little extra virgin olive oil

Salt

Directions:

Peel the potatoes and cut. Cut with match-sized mandolin, potatoes with a cane but very thin.

Wash and immerse in water 30 minutes.

Drain and dry well.

Add a little oil and stir so that the oil permeates well in all the potatoes.

Go to the basket of the air fryer and distribute well.

Select 1600C, 10 minutes.

Take out the basket; shake so that the potatoes take off. Let the potato tender. If it is not, leave 5 more minutes.

Place the steaks on top of the potatoes.

Select 1600C, 10 minutes and 180 degrees 5 minutes again.

Nutrition: Calories: 136Fat: 3.41g Carbohydrates: 0g Protein: 20.99g Sugar: 0

11   Homemade Flamingos

Preparation time: 10 minutes

Cooking time: 30 minutes

Servings: 4

Ingredients:

400g of very thin sliced pork fillets c / n

2 boiled and chopped eggs

100g chopped Serrano ham

1 beaten egg

Breadcrumbs

Directions:

Make a roll with the pork fillets. Introduce half-cooked egg and Serrano ham. So that the roll does not lose its shape, fasten with a string or chopsticks.

Pass the rolls through beaten egg and then through the breadcrumbs until it forms a good layer.

Preheat the air fryer a few minutes at 180° C.

Insert the rolls in the basket and set the timer for about 8 minutes at 180o C.

Nutrition: Calories: 482 Fat: 23.41 Carbohydrates: 0g Protein: 16.59 Sugar: 0g Cholesterol: 173gm

12   Braised Lamb With Vegetables

Preparation time: 10 minutes

Cooking time: 30 minutes

Servings: 6

Ingredients:

Salt and pepper to taste

2 ½ lb. boneless lamb leg, trimmed and sliced into cubes

1 tablespoon olive oil

1 onion, chopped

1 carrot, chopped

14 oz. canned diced tomatoes

1 cup low-sodium beef broth

1 tablespoon fresh rosemary, chopped

4 cloves garlic, minced

1 cup pearl onions

1 cup baby turnips, peeled and sliced into wedges

1 ½ cups baby carrots

1 ½ cups peas

2 tablespoons fresh parsley, chopped

Directions:

Sprinkle salt and pepper on both sides of the lamb.

Pour oil in a deep skillet.

Cook the lamb for 6 minutes.

Transfer lamb to a plate.

Add onion and carrot.

Cook for 3 minutes.

Stir in the tomatoes, broth, rosemary and garlic.

Simmer for 5 minutes.

Add the lamb back to the skillet.

Reduce heat to low.

Simmer for 1 hour and 15 minutes.

Add the pearl onion, baby carrot and baby turnips.

Simmer for 30 minutes.

Add the peas.

Cook for 1 minute.

Garnish with parsley before serving.

Nutrition: Calories 420 Total Fat 14 g Saturated Fat 4 g Cholesterol 126 mg Sodium 529 mg Total Carbohydrate 16 g Dietary Fiber 4 g Total Sugars 7 g Protein 43 g Potassium 988 mg

13   Beef With Broccoli

Preparation time: 10 minutes

Cooking time: 30 minutes

Servings: 4

Ingredients:

2 tablespoons olive oil, divided

2 garlic cloves, minced

1 pound beef sirloin steak, trimmed and sliced into thin strips

¼ cup low-sodium chicken broth

2 teaspoons fresh ginger, grated

1 tablespoon ground flax seeds

½ teaspoon red pepper flakes, crushed

Salt and ground black pepper, as required

1 large carrot, peeled and sliced thinly

2 cups broccoli florets

1 medium scallion, sliced thinly

Directions:

In a large skillet, heat 1 tablespoon of oil over medium-high heat and sauté the garlic for about 1 minute.

Add the beef and cook for about 4-5 minutes or until browned.

With a slotted spoon, transfer the beef into a bowl.

Remove the excess liquid from skillet.

In a bowl, add the broth, ginger, flax seeds, red pepper flakes, salt and black pepper.

In the same skillet, heat remaining oil over medium heat.

Add the carrot, broccoli and ginger mixture and cook for about 3-4 minutes or until desired doneness.

Stir in beef and scallion and cook for about 3-4 minutes.

Meal Prep Tip: Transfer the beef mixture into a large bowl and set aside to cool. Divide the mixture into 4 containers evenly. Cover the containers and refrigerate for 1-2 days. Reheat in the microwave before serving.

Nutrition: Calories 211 Total Fat 14.9 g Saturated Fat 3.9 g Cholesterol 101 mg Total Carbs 6.9 g Sugar 1.9 g Fiber 2.4 g Sodium 108 mg Potassium 706 mg Protein 36.5 g

14   Scrambled Eggs With Sausage

Preparation time: 10 minutes

Cooking time: 30 minutes

Servings: 2

Ingredients:

2 eggs

¼ cup cherry tomatoes

1 oz. turkey sausage, cooked and sliced

1 whole-grain muffin, halved and toasted

What you will need from the store cupboard:

2 tablespoons chicken broth

2 tablespoons low-fat Cheddar cheese, shredded

Ground black pepper

Cooking spray

Directions:

Apply cooking spray on your skillet.

Preheat over medium temperature.

Whisk together the broth, black pepper and eggs in a bowl.

Stir the sliced sausage in.

Now pour in the egg mixture.

Cook over medium temperature. Don't stir till you see the mixture starting to set around the edges and at the bottom.

Lift the fold the egg mix with a spoon or spatula. The uncooked part should flow below.

Keep cooking on medium till it is almost set.

Now add the cheese and tomatoes.

Cook for a minute more.

Serve over the toasted muffin halves.

Nutrition: Calories 198, Carbohydrates 16g, Fiber 2g, Cholesterol 231mg, Sugar 1g, Fat 9g, Protein 14g

---

Seafood

15   Air Fryer Fish & Chips

Preparation time: 10 minutes

Cooking Time:35 minutes

Servings: 4

Ingredients

4 cups of any fish fillet

flour: 1/4 cup

Whole wheat breadcrumbs: one cup

One egg

Oil: 2 tbsp.

Potatoes

Salt: 1 tsp.

Directions:

Cut the potatoes in fries. Then coat with oil and salt.

Cook in the air fryer for 20 minutes at 400 F, toss the fries halfway through.

In the meantime, coat fish in flour, then in the whisked egg, and finally in breadcrumbs mix.

Place the fish in the air fryer and let it cook at 330F for 15 minutes.

Flip it halfway through, if needed.

Serve with tartar sauce and salad green.

Nutrition: Calories: 409kcal | Carbohydrates: 44g | Protein: 30g | Fat: 11g |

16   Grilled Salmon with Lemon

Preparation time: 10 minutes

Cooking Time:20 minutes

Servings: 4

Ingredients

Olive oil: 2 tablespoons

Two Salmon fillets

Lemon juice

Water: 1/3 cup

Gluten-free light soy sauce: 1/3 cup

Honey: 1/3 cup

Scallion slices

Cherry tomato

Freshly ground black pepper, garlic powder, kosher salt to taste

Directions:

Season salmon with pepper and salt

In a bowl, mix honey, soy sauce, lemon juice, water, oil. Add salmon in this marinade and let it rest for least two hours.

Let the air fryer preheat at 180°C

Place fish in the air fryer and cook for 8 minutes.

Move to a dish and top with scallion slices.

Nutrition: Cal 211 | fat 9g | protein 15g | carbs 4.9g

17   Air-Fried Fish Nuggets

Preparation time: 15 minutes

Cooking Time:10 minutes

Servings: 4

Ingredients

Fish fillets in cubes: 2 cups(skinless)

1 egg, beaten

Flour: 5 tablespoons

Water: 5 tablespoons

Kosher salt and pepper to taste

Breadcrumbs mix

Smoked paprika: 1 tablespoon

Whole wheat breadcrumbs: ¼ cup

Garlic powder: 1 tablespoon

Directions:

Season the fish cubes with kosher salt and pepper.

In a bowl, add flour and gradually add water, mixing as you add.

Then mix in the egg. And keep mixing but do not over mix.

Coat the cubes in batter, then in the breadcrumb mix. Coat well

Place the cubes in a baking tray and spray with oil.

Let the air fryer preheat to 200 C.

Place cubes in the air fryer and cook for 12 minutes or until well cooked and golden brown.

Serve with salad greens.

Nutrition: Cal 184.2 | Protein: 19g | Total Fat: 3.3 g | Net Carb: 10g

18   Garlic Rosemary Grilled Prawns

Preparation time: 5 minutes

Cooking Time:10 minutes

Servings: 2

Ingredients

Melted butter: 1/2 tbsp.

Green capsicum: slices

Eight prawns

Rosemary leaves

Kosher salt& freshly ground black pepper

3-4 cloves of minced garlic

Directions:

In a bowl, mix all the ingredients and marinate the prawns in it for at least 60 minutes or more

Add two prawns and two slices of capsicum on each skewer.

Let the air fryer preheat to 180 C.

Cook for 5-6 minutes. Then change the temperature to 200 C and cook for another minute.

Serve with lemon wedges.

Nutrition: Cal 194 | Fat: 10g | Carbohydrates: 12g | protein: 26g

19   Air-Fried Crumbed Fish

Preparation time: 10 minutes

Cooking Time:12 minutes

Servings: 2

Ingredients

Four fish fillets

Olive oil: 4 tablespoons

One egg beaten

Whole wheat breadcrumbs: ¼ cup

Directions:

Let the air fryer preheat to 180 C.

In a bowl, mix breadcrumbs with oil. Mix well

First, coat the fish in the egg mix (egg mix with water) then in the breadcrumb mix. Coat well

Place in the air fryer, let it cook for 10-12 minutes.

Serve hot with salad green and lemon.

Nutrition: 254 Cal | fat 12.7g | carbohydrates10.2g | protein 15.5g.

Poultry

20   Spicy Mixed Greens

Preparation time: 10 minutes

Cooking time: 30 minutes

Servings: 6

Ingredients:

2 medium onions, chopped

1 pound mustard leaves, rinsed

1 pound fresh spinach, rinsed

2 tablespoons olive oil

4 garlic cloves, minced

1 (2-inch) piece fresh ginger, minced

1 teaspoon ground cumin

1 teaspoon ground coriander ½ teaspoon red chili powder

½ teaspoon ground turmeric

Salt and ground black pepper, as required

Directions:

In the Instant Pot, place oil and press "Sauté". Now add the onion, garlic, ginger, and spices and cook for about 2-3 minutes.

Add the greens and cook for about 2 minutes.

Press "Cancel" and stir well.

Close the lid and place the pressure valve to "Seal" position.

Press "Manual" and cook under "High Pressure" for about 4 minutes.

Press "Cancel" and allow a "Natural" release.

Open the lid and with an immersion blender, puree the mixture until smooth.

Serve immediately.

Nutrition: Calories: 98, Fats: 5.3g, Carbs: 11g, Sugar: 3.2g, Proteins: 4.8g, Sodium: 110mg

21   Spinach Stuffed Chicken Breast

Preparation time: 10 minutes

Cooking time: 30 minutes

Servings: 4

Ingredients:

4 chicken breasts

4 artichoke heart, chopped

4 teaspoons chopped sundried tomato

2 teaspoons minced garlic

¼ teaspoon ground black pepper

1 teaspoon curry powder

1 teaspoon paprika

20 basil leaves, chopped

4-ounce low-fat mozzarella cheese, chopped

1 cup water

Directions:

Place artichoke heart in a bowl, add tomato, garlic, basil, and mozzarella cheese and stir until mixed.

Cut each chicken breast halfway through and then season chicken with salt, black pepper, curry powder, and paprika. Stuff chicken with artichoke mixture and close the filling with chicken using a toothpick.

Plugin instant pot, insert the inner pot, pour in water, then insert steamer basket and place stuffed chicken breasts on it.

Shut the instant pot with its lid, turn the pressure knob to seal the pot, press the 'manual' button, then press the 'timer' to set the cooking time to 15 minutes and cook at high pressure, instant pot will take 5 minutes or more for building its inner pressure.

When the timer beeps, press 'cancel' button and do natural pressure release for 10 minutes and then do quick pressure release until pressure nob drops down.

Open the instant pot, transfer stuffed chicken to plates and serve.

Nutrition: Calories: 262 Cal, Carbs: 8.5 g, Fat: 4.1 g, Protein: 46.1 g, Fiber: 2.4 g.

22　Chicken With Salsa

Preparation time: 10 minutes

Cooking time: 30 minutes

Servings: 4

Ingredients:

4 (6-ounce) boneless, skinless frozen chicken breasts

1 cup homemade tomato puree

1 cup mild salsa

¼ cup low-fat Parmesan cheese, grated

3 tablespoons fresh lime juice

Ground black pepper, as required

Directions:

In the pot of Instant Pot, place all ingredients except cheese and mix well.

Close the lid and place the pressure valve to "Seal" position.

Press "Manual" and cook under "High Pressure" for about 12 minutes.

Meanwhile, preheat the oven to broiler. Grease a baking dish.

Press "Cancel" and carefully allow a "Quick" release.

Open the lid and with tongs, transfer the chicken breasts into the prepared baking dish.

Now, Press "Sauté" of Instant Pot and cook for about 2-3 minutes or until desired thickness of mixture.

Press "Cancel" and pour the sauce over chicken breasts.

Sprinkle with cheese and broil for about 4-5 minutes.

Serve hot.

Nutrition: Calories: 381, Fats: 14.2g, Carbs: 8.7g, Sugar: 4.8g, Proteins: 52.2g, Sodium: 600mg

23   Rosemary Lemon Chicken

Preparation time: 10 minutes

Cooking time: 30 minutes

Servings: 4

Ingredients:

1 kg chicken breast halves

1 lemon, peeled and sliced into rounds

1/2 orange, peeled and sliced into rounds, or to taste

3 cloves roasted garlic, or to taste

salt and ground black pepper to taste

1 1/2 tablespoons olive oil, or to taste

1 1/2 teaspoons agave syrup, or to taste (optional)

1/4 cup water

2 sprigs fresh rosemary, stemmed, or to taste

Directions:

Place chicken in the Instant Pot. Add lemon, orange, and garlic; season with salt and pepper. Drizzle olive oil and agave syrup (if using) on top. Add water and rosemary. Put the lid on the cooker and Lock in place.

Select the "Meat" and "Stew" settings for High pressure, and cook for 14 minutes. Allow pressure to release naturally, about 20 minutes.

Nutrition: Calories 325 Fat 5 g Carbohydrates 20 g Sugar 2 g Protein 10 g Cholesterol 33 mg

24   Ginger Flavored Chicken

Preparation time: 10 minutes

Cooking time: 30 minutes

Servings: 6

Ingredients:

1 kg boneless, skinless chicken breasts (frozen OR thawed)

6 tablespoons soy sauce

3 tablespoons rice vinegar

1/2 tablespoon honey

3 tablespoons water, broth, or orange juice

2 tablespoons chopped fresh ginger

6 cloves garlic, minced

3 teaspoons corn starch

Directions:

Place chicken breasts in Instant Pot.

In a small mixing bowl, whisk together: vinegar, soy sauce, honey, water, ginger and garlic. Pour mixture over chicken and coat evenly.

Secure lid on Instant Pot and cook at High pressure for 15 minutes. When the meat is cooked, release steam.

Remove chicken breasts and place on a cutting board. Bring remaining sauce in pan up to a simmer (use the Saute feature on an electric cooker). Combine cornstarch with 3 teaspoons cold water and then pour mixture into pan. Simmer until sauce is thickened and the turn off heat.

Shred chicken and return to pot with sauce.

Nutrition: Calories 313 Fat 25.6 g Carbohydrates 15.6 g Sugar 7 g Protein 8 g Cholesterol 36 mg

25   Crockpot Slow Cooker Tex-mex Chicken

Preparation time: 10 minutes

Cooking time: 30 minutes

Servings: 6

Ingredients:

4 tablespoons cup water

1 teaspoon ground cumin

1 lb boneless chicken thighs, visible fat removed, rinsed, and patted dry

1 (10 oz) can diced tomatoes and green chilies

1 (16 oz) package frozen onion and pepper strips, thawed

Directions:

Spray a skillet with cooking spray and turn heat flame on.

Place chicken thighs into the skillet and cook each side until browned over medium heat. Once browned, take out from the skillet.

To the same skillet, add peppers and onions and cook until tender.

Transfer cooked peppers and onions into 4-to 5-quart Crock-Pot slow cooker followed by chicken thighs on top.

Place tomatoes along with 4 tablespoons of water over chicken. Cook for about 4 hours on Low.

Add 1 teaspoon ground cumin and cook further for half an hour.

Once done, take it out and serve right away!

Nutrition: 121 calories; 3.2 g fat; 6.4 g total carbs; 16 g protein

26   Slow-cooker Chicken Fajita Burritos

Preparation time: 10 minutes

Cooking time: 30 minutes

Servings: 8

Ingredients:

1 teaspoon cumin

1 cup cheddar cheese + 2 tablespoons reduced-fat, shredded

1 lb. chicken strips, skinless and boneless

8 large low-carb tortillas

1 green pepper, sliced

1 can (15 oz) black beans, rinsed and drained

1 red pepper, sliced

1/3 cup water

1 medium onion, sliced

½ cup salsa

1 tablespoon chili powder

1 teaspoon garlic powder

Directions:

Place strips of chicken breast in a slow-cooker.

Top chicken with all ingredients mentioned above except for cheese and tortillas. Cover the cooker and cook for approximately 6 hours, until done.

Shred chicken with a fork.

Serve half cup of chicken on each tortilla along with the bean mixture.

Finish with 2 tablespoons of shredded cheese, then fold tortilla into a burrito.

Nutrition: 250 calories; 7 g fat; 31 g total carbs; 28 g protei

Soup and Stews

27   Lamb Stew

Preparation time: 15 Minutes

Cooking time: 35 minutes

Servings: 2

Ingredients:

1lb diced lamb shoulder

1lb chopped winter vegetables

1 cup low sodium vegetable broth

1tbsp yeast extract

1tbsp star anise spice mix

Directions:

Mix all the ingredients in your Instant Pot.

Cook on Stew for 35 minutes.

Release the pressure naturally.

Nutrition: Calories: 320; Carbs: 10; Sugar: 2; Fat: 8; Protein: 42; GL: 3

28   Irish Stew

Preparation time: 15 Minutes

Cooking time: 35 minutes

Servings: 2

Ingredients:

1.5lb diced lamb shoulder

1lb chopped vegetables

1 cup low sodium beef broth

3 minced onions

1tbsp ghee

Directions:

Mix all the ingredients in your Instant Pot.

Cook on Stew for 35 minutes.

Release the pressure naturally.

Nutrition: Calories: 330; Carbs: 9; Sugar: 2; Fat: 12; Protein: 49; GL: 3

29   Sweet And Sour Soup

Preparation time: 15 Minutes

Cooking time: 35 minutes

Servings: 2

Ingredients:

1lb cubed chicken breast

1lb chopped vegetables

1 cup low carb sweet and sour sauce

0.5 cup diabetic marmalade

Directions:

Mix all the ingredients in your Instant Pot.

Cook on Stew for 35 minutes.

Release the pressure naturally.

30   Meatball Stew

Preparation time: 15 Minutes

Cooking time: 25 minutes

Servings: 2

Ingredients:

1lb sausage meat

2 cups chopped tomato

1 cup chopped vegetables

2tbsp Italian seasonings

1tbsp vegetable oil

Directions:

Roll the sausage into meatballs.

Put the Instant Pot on Sauté and fry the meatballs in the oil until brown.

Mix all the ingredients in your Instant Pot.

Cook on Stew for 25 minutes.

Release the pressure naturally.

Nutrition: Calories: 300; Carbs: 4; Sugar: 1; Fat: 12; Protein: 40; GL: 2

31 Kebab Stew

Preparation time: 15 Minutes

Cooking time: 35 minutes

Servings: 2

Ingredients:

1lb cubed, seasoned kebab meat

1lb cooked chickpeas

1 cup low sodium vegetable broth

1tbsp black pepper

Directions:

Mix all the ingredients in your Instant Pot.

Cook on Stew for 35 minutes.

Release the pressure naturally.

Nutrition: Calories: 290; Carbs: 22; Sugar: 4; Fat: 10; Protein: 34; GL: 6

32 French Onion Soup

Preparation time: 35 Minutes

Cooking time: 35 minutes

Servings: 2

Ingredients:

6 onions, chopped finely

2 cups vegetable broth

2tbsp oil

2tbsp Gruyere

Directions:

Place the oil in your Instant Pot and cook the onions on Sauté until soft and brown.

Mix all the ingredients in your Instant Pot.

Cook on Stew for 35 minutes.

Release the pressure naturally.

 Nutrition: Calories: 110; Carbs: 8; Sugar: 3; Fat: 10; Protein: 3; GL: 4

Salads, Sauces, Dressings & Dips

33   Almond Pasta Salad

Preparation Time: 10 minutes

Cooking Time: 10 minutes

Servings: 6

Ingredients:

1 lb. elbow macaroni, cooked

1/2 cup sun-dried tomatoes, diced

1 (15 oz.) can make whole artichokes, diced

1 orange bell pepper, diced

3 green onions, sliced

2 tablespoons basil, sliced

2 oz. slivered almonds

Dressing:

1 garlic clove, minced

1 tablespoon Dijon mustard

1 tablespoon raw honey

1/4 cup white balsamic vinegar

1/3 cup olive oil

Directions:

Preheat the oven to 350 degrees F.

Lay the almonds on a baking sheet and bake until golden brown.

Cook the pasta as the package instruction.

Move to a serving bowl and start tossing all the ingredients.

Mix well and serve.

Nutrition:

Calories 260

Fat 7.7g

Sodium 143mg

Phosphorus 39mg

Potassium 585mg

Carbohydrate 41.4g

Protein 9.6g

34   Pineapple Berry Salad

Preparation Time: 10 minutes

Cooking Time: 5 minutes

Servings: 4

Ingredients:

4 cups pineapple, peeled and cubed

3 cups strawberries, chopped

1/4 cup honey

1/2 cup basil leaves

1 tablespoon lemon zest

1/2 cup blueberries

Directions:

Prepare a salad bowl.

Put all the ingredients.

Mix well and serve.

Nutrition:

Calories 128

Fat 0.6g

Sodium 3mg

Phosphorous 151mg

Potassium 362mg

Carbohydrate 33.1g

Protein 1.8g

35   Cabbage Pear Salad

Preparation Time: 15 minutes

Cooking Time: 1 hour

Servings: 6

Ingredients:

2 scallions, chopped

2 cups finely shredded green cabbage

1 cup finely shredded red cabbage

½ red bell pepper, boiled and chopped

½ cup chopped cilantro

2 celery stalks, chopped

1 Asian pear, cored and grated

1/4 cup olive oil

Juice of 1 lime

Zest of 1 lime

1 teaspoon granulated sugar

Directions:

In a mixing bowl, add cabbages, scallions, celery, pear, red pepper, and cilantro.

Combine to mix well with each other.

Take another mixing bowl; add olive oil, lime juice, lime zest, and sugar. Mix well with each other.

Add dressing over and toss well.

Refrigerate for 1 hour; serve chilled.

Nutrition:

Calories: 128

Fat: 8g

Sodium: 57mg

Potassium: 149mg

Phosphorus: 25mg

Carbohydrates: 2g

Protein: 6g

36   Vegetables with Apple Juice

Preparation Time: 10 minutes

Cooking Time: 50 minutes

Servings: 4

Ingredients:

3 tablespoons olive oil

3 cups apple juice

1 1/4 pounds turnips

1 1/4 pounds carrots

1 1/4 pounds cauliflower

Salt and pepper to taste

Directions:

Boil apple juice in a large saucepan until reduced to 3/4 cup, about 30 minutes. Whisk in olive oil.

Preheat oven to 425 degrees F.

Peel and cut vegetables into 1/2-inch pieces. Divide between 2 roasting pans.

Pour apple juice mixture over vegetables. Sprinkle with salt and pepper. Toss to coat.

Roast until vegetables are tender and golden, occasionally stirring, about 40 minutes.

Nutrition:

Calories 91

Fat 4.4g

Sodium 19mg

Potassium 215mg

Phosphorus 150 mg

Carbohydrate 13.3g

Dietary Fiber 1.5g

Protein 0.5g

Dessert and Snacks

37   Cranberry Pound Cake

Preparation time: 10 minutes
Cooking time: 15 minutes
Servings: 12
Ingredients
2 cups all-purpose flour
1 1/4 teaspoons baking powder
1/2 teaspoon baking soda 3 tablespoons butter, softened
1/2 cup Splenda Sugar Blend for Baking
 2 eggs
1/4 teaspoon orange extract (optional)
2/3 cup plain nonfat yogurt 2 cups fresh cranberries
1/4 cup water or 1/4 cup orange juice
1 1/2 teaspoons orange zest, finely grated
Directions
Preheat oven to 350F. Prepare bundt or tube pan with a light
coat of cooking spray.

In a medium bowl, sift together the flour, baking soda and baking powder.

In a large bowl, cream the butter with an electric mixer. Add Splenda blend and beat until pale, light and fluffy. Add the eggs, one at a time, mixing after each addition for a total of two or three minutes. If want more orange flavor, mix in the orange extract at this step.

Mix together the yogurt and water or orange juice.

Add in the cranberries, folding in to distribute throughout the batter.

Pour batter into the prepare tube pan and bake for 40 minutes or until an inserted toothpick comes out clean.

Cool cake in pan for 10 minutes until turning onto cake rack or plate.

Nutrition: 161 Calories; 4g fat; 27g Carbohydrates; 4g Protein; per 1/12 of recipe

38   Diabetic Friendly Carrot Cake

Preparation time: 10 minutes

Cooking time: 15 minutes

Servings: 12

Ingredients

2 cups shredded carrots

4 ounces unsweetened crushed pineapple with juice

3/4 cup Splenda brown sugar blend 2 teaspoons vanilla

extract

2 cups white whole wheat flour

1/2 teaspoon baking soda 2 teaspoons baking powder

1 cup unsweetened applesauce

3 egg whites

1/4 teaspoon salt 1 teaspoon ground cinnamon

1 container sugar-free white frosting (16 oz)

Directions

Preheat oven to 350 F. Coat a 9 x 13inch baking dish with cooking spray.

In a large bowl, combine carrots, pineapple, brown sugar blend, applesauce, egg whites, and vanilla. Add remaining ingredients except frosting mix well. Spread batter in baking dish.

Bake for 25 to 30 minutes, or until wooden toothpick inserted in center comes out clean. Let cool, then spread frosting over cake and serve.

Nutritional Information Per 1/16 of Recipe: Calories 119; Total Fat 4 g; Saturated Fat 1 g; Cholesterol 0 mg; Carbohydrates 22 g; Fiber 3 g; Protein 2 g; Sodium 143 mg

39   Cinnamon Oatmeal Cookies

Preparation time: 10 minutes

Cooking time: 45 minutes

Servings: 12

Ingredients

1 cup quick-cooking oats

3/4 cup whole wheat flour

2 teaspoons ground cinnamon

1 1/2 teaspoon baking powder

1/4 teaspoon salt

2 tablespoons margarine, melted and cooled

1 egg

1 teaspoon vanilla extract

1/2 cup sugar-free maple syrup

Glaze

2 tablespoons reduced-fat cream cheese, softened

2 teaspoons low fat milk

1 teaspoon vanilla extract

2 tablespoons confectioners' sugar

Directions

Preheat oven to 325 F. Coat a baking sheet with cooking spray.

In a medium bowl, combine oats, flour, baking powder, cinnamon, and salt.

In a small bowl, mix margarine, vanilla and eggstir in honey. Add to flour mixture and mix well. Stir in chocolate chips. Refrigerate dough 30 minutes, then shape into 14 balls and flatten slightly. Place on baking sheet about 2 inches apart. Bake 10 to 12 minutes, or until brown around the edges. Let cool 5 minutes, then remove to a wire rack to cool completely.

Nutrition: 64 calories; 2.5 g fat; 1 g fiber; 9 g carbohydrates; 2 g protein

40   Crustless Cheesecake

Preparation time: 10 minutes

Cooking time: 35 minutes

Servings: 12

Ingredients

2 (8-ounce) packages reduced-fat cream cheese, softened

2/3 cup Splenda

3 eggs

1/2 teaspoon vanilla extract

1/4 teaspoon fresh lemon juice

Topping:

2 cups (16 ounces) reduced-fat sour cream

3 tablespoons sugar

1 teaspoon vanilla extract
1/4 teaspoon fresh lemon juice

Directions
Preheat oven to 325 F. Coat a 9-inch pie plate with cooking spray.
In a large bowl, combine cream cheese and 2/3 cup Splenda; beat well. Beat in eggs, one at a time. Beat in 1/2 teaspoon vanilla and 1/4 teaspoon lemon juice. Spoon mixture into pie plate.
Bake 45 to 50 minutes, until golden. Remove from oven and let cool 10 to 15 minutes.
In another large bowl, combine topping ingredients. Spread over top of cheesecake and bake 10 minutes. Let cool then refrigerate overnight or at least 4 hours before serving.
Nutrition: 246 calories; 14 g fat; 0 g fiber; 23 g carbohydrates; 7 g protein; per 1/10 of recipe

41   Apple Cake

Preparation time: 10 minutes

Cooking time: 40 minutes

Servings: 10

Ingredients:

1 tbsp vegetable oil

2 large Granny Smith apples, peeled and halved; cut 8 thin slices (set aside) and chop the remainder

2 tsp ground cinnamon

1 ¼ cup all-purpose flour

¾ tsp baking powder

½ tsp baking soda

½ cup sweetener

½ cup light buttery spread

2 eggs

¾ cup plain nonfat yogurt or low-fat buttermilk

1 tbsp confectioner's sweetener

Directions:

Preheat the oven to 350°F.

Line an 8-inch cake pan with parchment paper.

Heat the oil and fry the chopped apples for a few minutes.

Toss the apples in cinnamon and continue to fry for a further 2 minutes. Set aside.

Cream the buttery spread with the sweetener until fluffy.

Add the eggs and mix well.

Fold in the yogurt, flour, baking powder, and soda.

Stir in the cooked apples.

Spoon the batter into the tin and arrange the apple slices on top.

Bake for 35 to 40 minutes. Test the cake with a skewer to ensure it's cooked through.

Cool the cake on a wire rack and dredge with confectioner's sweetener.

Nutrition: Calories 105, Total Carbs 29g, Net Carbs 28g, Fat 7g, Protein 4g, Sodium 185mg

42   Diabetic Sour Cream Coffee Cake

Preparation time: 25 minutes

Cooking time: 1 hour

Servings: 16

Ingredients:

1/3 cup walnuts, chopped

1½ tsp cinnamon

1 cup sweetener

3 cups all-purpose flour

1 tsp baking soda

2 tsp grated lemon zest

1 tsp almond extract

2 eggs

1 egg white

1/3 cup canola oil

½ cup plain nonfat yogurt

¼ cup unsweetened applesauce

1½ cup nonfat sour cream

Directions:

Preheat the oven to 350°F.

Spray a 12-cup Bundt pan with nonstick cooking spray. Set aside.

Mix the walnuts, cinnamon, and a quarter of the sweetener in a small bowl and set aside.

Mix the wet ingredients in a large bowl with an electric mixer.

Add the flour, the remaining sweetener, baking soda, and lemon zest and mix well.

Pour the batter into the pan.

Sprinkle over the sweetener -walnut mixture.

Bake for 1 hour. Use a skewer to test the cake is cooked through.

Cool on a wire rack before removing from the pan.

Nutrition: Calories 225, Total Carbs 32g, Net Carbs 31g, Fat 7g, Protein 6g, Sodium 110mg

43   Light Lemon Vanilla Sponge Cake

Preparation time: 25 minutes

Cooking time: 1 hour

Servings: 14

Ingredients:

Nonstick cooking spray

½ cup canola oil

1¼ cup sweetener

2 whole eggs

4 egg whites

1 cup nonfat lemon yogurt

Grated zest and juice of 1 lemon

1 tbsp vanilla

2¼ cup all-purpose flour

1 tsp baking powder

½ tsp baking soda

¼ tsp cream of tartar

pinch salt

¼ cup confectioners' sweetener

Directions:

Preheat the oven to 325°F.

Spray a 9-inch round cake pan with cooking spray.

Mix all the wet ingredients in a medium bowl until well blended.

Combine the dry ingredients and lemon zest and then fold into the wet mixture.

Pour the batter into the prepared tin and bake for 1 hour.

Test the cake with a skewer to ensure its cooked through.

Leave to cool on a wire rack, then dredge with confectioner's sweetener after removing from the pan.

Nutrition: Calories 250, Total Carbs 38g, Net Carbs 38g, Fat 9g, Protein 4g, Sodium 105mg

44   Butterscotch Brownies

Preparation time: 10 minutes

Cooking time: 15 minutes

Servings: 12

Ingredients

1 cup margarine

3 cups Splenda brown sugar blend

1 cup liquid egg substitute

3 tablespoons vanilla extract

1 1/2 cup all-purpose flour

3 teaspoons baking powder

1 1/2 cup almonds, chopped

Directions

Preheat oven to 350 degrees F. Lightly spray a 9-x 13-inch baking pan with cooking spray.

Cream margarine and sugar together until fluffy. Add eggs, one at a time, scraping bowl between each addition. Add the rest of the ingredients and mix until smooth.

Spread the mixture into the baking pan. Bake 30 to 40 minutes, or until a toothpick inserted into the center comes out clean.

Nutrition: 170 calories; 12 g fat; 4 g fiber; 11 g carbohydrates; 4 g protein; per 1/16 of recipe

45   Pecan Squares

Preparation time: 10 minutes

Cooking time: 25 minutes

Servings: 12

Ingredients

2 1/4 cups all-purpose flour

1 cup packed Splenda brown sugar substitute

1/4 cup (1/2 stick) light butter, softened

1 (15-ounce) can pears in light syrup, chopped, juice reserved

1/2 cup egg substitute

1 teaspoon vanilla extract

2 teaspoons baking soda

1 teaspoon salt

3 tablespoons chopped pecans

Directions

Preheat the oven to 350F. Coat a 9 x 13-inch baking dish with cooking spray.

In a large bowl, using an electric mixer, beat the flour, brown sugar, butter, reserved pear juice, egg substitute, vanilla extract, baking soda, and salt for 2 minutes, or until smooth. Stir in the chopped pears then pour the mixture into the baking dish; top with the chopped pecans.

Bake for 25-30 minutes, or until a wooden toothpick inserted in the center comes out clean. Allow to cool completely then cut into squares and serve or store in an airtight container until ready to serve.

Nutrition: 232 calories; 13 g fat; 2 g fiber; 27 g carbohydrates; 4 g protein; per 1/20 of recipe

46   Double Chocolate Biscotti

Preparation time: 10 Minutes

Cooking time: 40 minutes

Servings: 27

Ingredients:

3 egg whites, divided

2 eggs

1 tbsp. orange zest

What you'll need from store cupboard:

2 cup flour

½ cup Splenda

½ cup almonds, toasted and chopped

1/3 cup cocoa, unsweetened

¼ cup mini chocolate chips

1 tsp vanilla

1 tsp instant coffee granules

1 tsp water

½ tsp salt

½ tsp baking soda

Nonstick cooking spray

Directions:

Heat oven to 350 degrees. Spray a large baking sheet with cooking spray.

In a large bowl, combine flour, Splenda, cocoa, salt, and baking soda.

In a small bowl, whisk the eggs, 2 egg whites, vanilla, and coffee. Let rest 3-4 minutes to dissolve the coffee.

Stir in the orange zest and add to dry Ingredients, stir to thoroughly combine. Fold in the nuts and chocolate chips. Divide dough in half and place on prepared pan. Shape each half into 14x1 ¾-inch rectangle.

Stir water and remaining egg white together. Brush over the top of the dough. Bake 20-25 minutes, or until firm to the touch. Cool on wire racks 5 minutes.

Transfer biscotti to a cutting board. Use a serrated knife to cut diagonally into ½-inch slice. Place cut side down on baking sheet and bake 5-7 minutes per side. Store in airtight container. Serving size is 2 pieces.

Nutrition: Calories 86 Total Carbs 13g Net Carbs 12g Protein 3g Fat 3g Sugar 5g Fiber 1g

47   Apple Mini Cakes

Preparation time: 10 Minutes

Cooking time: 40 minutes

Servings: 2

Ingredients:

1 medium apple, peeled and diced, into bite-sized pieces

18g granulated sugar

18g unsalted butter

2g ground cinnamon

1g ground nutmeg

1g ground allspice

1 sheet prefabricated cake dough

1 beaten egg

5 ml of milk

Directions:

Put diced apples, granulated sugar, butter, cinnamon, nutmeg, and allspice in a medium saucepan or in a skillet over medium-low heat.

Simmer for 2 minutes and remove from heat.

Allow the apples to cool, discovered at room temperature for 30 minutes.

Cut the cake dough into circles of 127 mm.

Add the filling to the center of each circle and use your finger to apply water to the outer ends. Some filler will be left unused.

Close the cake cut a small opening at the top.

Preheat the air fryer for a few minutes and set the temperature to 175°C.

Mix the eggs and milk and spread the mixture on each foot.

Place the cakes in the preheated air fryer and cook at 175°C for 10 minutes until the cakes are golden brown.

Nutrition: (Nutrition per Serving)Calories: 185 Fat: 11Carbohydrates: 38g Protein: 5g Sugar: 20gCholesterol: 11mg

48   Orange Oatmeal Cookies

Preparation time: 10 Minutes

Cooking time: 40 minutes

Servings: 18 (2 Cookies Per Serving)

Ingredients:

1 orange, zested and juiced

½ cup margarine

1 egg white

1 tbsp. orange juice

What you'll need from the store cupboard

1 cup whole wheat pastry flour

1 cup oats

¼ cup stevia

¼ cup dark brown sugar substitute

¼ cup applesauce, unsweetened

1/3 cup wheat bran

½ tsp baking soda

½ tsp cream of tartar

¼ tsp cinnamon

Directions:

Heat oven to 350 degrees. Line two cookie sheets with parchment paper.

In a medium mixing bowl, cream butter. Gradually add the sugars and beat 2 -3 minutes.

Add egg white and applesauce and beat just to combine.

Sift the dry Ingredients together in a large mixing bowl. Add the wet Ingredients, the orange juice, and the zest.

Drop the dough by tablespoons onto the prepared cookie sheets. Bake 10 minutes, or until the bottoms are brown. Cool on wire rack. Store in an airtight container.

Nutrition: Calories 129 Total Carbs 17g Net Carbs 16g Protein 2g Fat 6g Sugar 8g Fiber 1g

49 Apple Pear & Pecan Dessert Squares

Preparation time: 10 Minutes

Cooking time: 40 minutes

Servings: 24

Ingredients:

1 Granny Smith apple, sliced, leave peel on

1 Red Delicious apple, sliced, leave peel on

1 ripe pear, sliced, leave peel on

3 eggs

½ cup plain fat-free yogurt

1 tbsp. lemon juice

1 tbsp. margarine

What you'll need from store cupboard:

1 package spice cake mix

1 ¼ cup water, divided

½ cup pecan pieces

1 tbsp. Splenda

1 tsp cinnamon

½ tsp vanilla

¼ tsp nutmeg

Nonstick cooking spray

Directions:

Heat oven to 350°F. Spray jelly-roll pan with nonstick cooking spray.

In a large bowl, beat cake mix, 1 cup water, eggs and yogurt until smooth. Pour into prepared pan and bake 20 minutes or it passes the toothpick test. Cool completely.

In a large nonstick skillet, over med-high heat, toast the pecans, stirring, about 2 minutes or until lightly browned. Remove to a plate.

Add the remaining ¼ cup water, sliced fruit, juice and spices to the skillet. Bring to a boil. Reduce heat to medium and cook 3 minutes or until fruit is tender crisp.

Remove from heat and stir in Splenda, margarine, vanilla, and pecans. Spoon evenly over cooled cake. Slice into 24 squares and serve.

Nutrition: Calories 130 Total Carbs 20g Net Carbs 19g Protein 2g Fat 5g Sugar 10g Fiber 1g

50   Mini Bread Puddings

Preparation time: 10 Minutes

Cooking time: 40 minutes

Servings: 12

Ingredients:

6 slices cinnamon bread, cut into cubes

1 ¼ cup skim milk

½ cup egg substitute

1 tbsp. margarine, melted

What you'll need from store cupboard

1/3 cup Splenda

1 tsp vanilla

1/8 tsp salt

1/8 tsp nutmeg

Directions:

Heat oven to 350°F. Line 12 medium-size muffin cups with paper baking cups.

In a large bowl, stir together milk, egg substitute, Splenda, vanilla, salt and nutmeg until combined. Add bread cubes and stir until moistened. Let rest 15 minutes.

Spoon evenly into prepared baking cups. Drizzle margarine evenly over the tops. Bake 30-35 minutes or until puffed and golden brown. Remove from oven and let cool completely.

Nutrition: Calories 105 Total Carbs 16 Net Carbs 15g Protein 4g Fat 2g Sugar 9g Fiber 1g

Conclusion

Diabetes can be managed and treated effectively, although the process of doing so requires knowledge, discipline, patience and passion. Your health and happiness does not have to drop along with your insulin and blood glucose levels. In fact, you can make your life even better if you learn as much as you can about how your body functions as a diabetic and follow a healthy lifestyle suitable for diabetics.

Most of the successful management of diabetes relies on the right food choices, and getting enough exercise. Diabetes is a long term condition which you will have to deal with for the rest of your life, but you can lead a full and active life when you are armed with the knowledge you need to understand and manage your condition.

Hypoglycemia is an ever present concern for diabetics. That's when the blood sugar levels drop dangerously low, and weight loss diets and too much exercise can cause a hypoglycemic incident. In fact, just about everything about diabetes revolves around blood glucose levels, so it's important that you understand how to keep these levels stable.

Diabetes in itself is not necessarily life-threatening, but there can be complications as a result of the condition and again, most of these complications can be attributed to fluctuating blood glucose levels, which can cause a lot of stress to the system. Most of the complications associated with diabetes – including diabetic neuropathies, retinal neuropathy, heart disease, high blood pressure and high cholesterol – can be prevented or controlled by keeping blood glucose levels within the healthy range.

Knowledge is power, so make sure you learn as much as possible about the treatment and management of diabetes, particularly how it affects you as an individual, because every diabetes journey is unique. What works for your friend or neighbor may not necessarily be the right thing for you.

Make friends with and make use of your health care providers, because they can help you to manage your condition effectively. They have seen all the complications and permutations, and they know how to address your concerns and help you through the bad spells and the down times. No matter how well you manage your diabetes, there will be times when nothing seems to go right, and you feel unwell, afraid and alone. The support of your family and your medical team will help you through those times.

Always wear your medical ID, and make sure that people you work with and socialize with know that you are diabetic, and what to do should you become ill. It's particularly important to notify the instructor if you attend an exercise class or the gym, so that they can take appropriate action to get you the treatment you need as quickly as possible should you have problems.

Above all, live your life as you want to, but always remember that you have diabetes and that there are adjustments you will need to make to your lifestyle if you are to stay fit and well. Treating and managing your diabetes will enable you to achieve the fit body and healthy lifestyle that everyone wants, whether or not they are diabetic. With the help of the tips and strategies in this book, you can start changing your life for the better right now.

Knowledge is power, so make sure you learn as much as possible about the treatment and management of diabetes, particularly how it affects you as an individual, because every diabetes journey is unique. What works for your friend or neighbor may not necessarily be the right thing for you. Make friends with and make use of your health care providers, because they can help you to manage your condition effectively. They have seen all the complications and permutations, and they know how to address your concerns and help you through the bad spells and the down times. No matter how well you manage your diabetes, there will be times when nothing seems to go right, and you feel unwell, afraid and alone. The support of your family and your medical team will help you through those times.

Always wear your medical ID, and make sure that people you work with and socialize with know that you are diabetic, and what to do should you become ill. It's particularly important to notify the instructor if you attend an exercise class or the gym, so that they can take appropriate action to get you the treatment you need as quickly as possible should you have problems.

Above all, live your life as you want to, but always remember that you have diabetes and that there are adjustments you will need to make to your lifestyle if you are to stay fit and well. Treating and managing your diabetes will enable you to achieve the fit body and healthy lifestyle that everyone wants, whether or not they are diabetic. With the help of the tips and strategies in this book, you can start changing your life for the better right now.

Why did I start this book? Having Type 1 diabetes will teach you a load of tough lessons. Only about ¼ of diabetics are Type 1. But I'm here to tell you, even though Type 1 is the most common type of diabetes, Type 2 diabetes can be almost as bad. I'm telling you this because I don't want you to get discouraged and give up.

Being diagnosed with the disease will bring some major changes in your lifestyle. From the time you are diagnosed with it, it would always be a constant battle with food. You need to become a lot more careful with your food choices and the quantity that you ate. Every meal will feel like a major effort. You will be planning every day for the whole week, well in advance. Depending upon the type of food you ate, you have to keep checking your blood sugar levels. You may get used to taking long breaks between meals and staying away from snacks between dinner and breakfast.

Food would be treated as a bomb like it can go off at any time. According to an old saying, "When the body gets too hot, then your body heads straight to the kitchen."

Managing diabetes can be a very, very stressful ordeal. There will be many times that you will mark your glucose levels down on a piece of paper like you are plotting graph lines or something. You will mix your insulin shots up and then stress about whether or not you are giving yourself the right dosage. You will always be over-cautious because it involves a LOT of math and a really fine margin of error. But now, those days are gone!

With the help of technology and books, you can stock your kitchen with the right foods, like meal plans, diabetic friendly dishes, etc. You can get an app that will even do the work for you. You can also people-watch on the internet and find the know-how to cook and eat right; you will always be a few meals away from certain disasters, like a plummeting blood sugar level. Always carry some sugar in your pocket. You won't have to experience the pangs of hunger but if you are unlucky, you will have to ration your food and bring along some simple low-calorie snacks with you.

This is the future of diabetes.

As you've reached the end of this book, you have gained complete control of your diabetes and this is just the beginning of your journey towards a better, healthier life. I hope I was able to inculcate some knowledge into you and make this adventure a little bit less of a struggle.

I would like to remind you that you're not alone in having to manage this disease and that nearly 85% of the new cases are 20 years old or younger.

Regardless of the length or seriousness of your diabetes, it can be managed! Take the information presented here and start with it!

Preparation is key to having a healthier and happier life.

It's helpful to remember that every tool at your disposal can help in some way.

CPSIA information can be obtained
at www.ICGtesting.com
Printed in the USA
BVHW041009150321
602551BV00006B/335